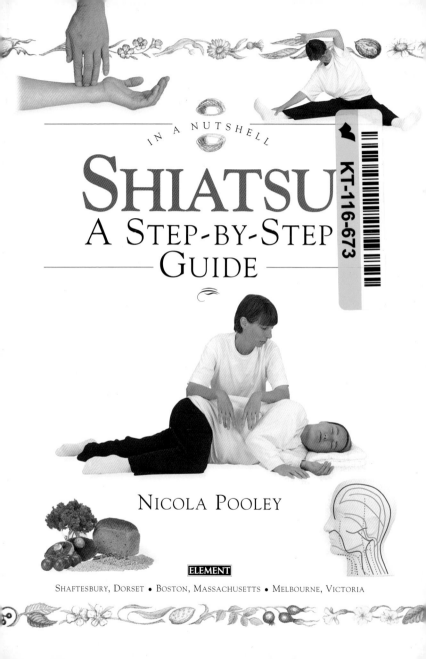

IN A NUTSHELL

SHIATSU
A STEP-BY-STEP
GUIDE

NICOLA POOLEY

ELEMENT

SHAFTESBURY, DORSET • BOSTON, MASSACHUSETTS • MELBOURNE, VICTORIA

© Element Books Limited 1998

First published in
Great Britain in 1998 by
ELEMENT BOOKS LIMITED
Shaftesbury,
Dorset SP7 9BP

Published in the USA in 1998 by
ELEMENT BOOKS INC
160 North Washington Street,
Boston MA 02114

Published in Australia in 1998 by
ELEMENT BOOKS LIMITED
and distributed by Penguin Australia Ltd
487 Maroondah Highway, Ringwood,
Victoria 3134

Reprinted September 1998 , March 1999

NOTE FROM THE PUBLISHER
Any information given in this book is
not intended to be taken as a replacement
for medical advice. Any person with
a condition requiring medical attention
should consult a qualified practitioner
or therapist.

Designed and created with
The Bridgewater Book Company Ltd

ELEMENT BOOKS LIMITED
Managing Editor Miranda Spicer
Senior Commissioning Editor Caro Ness
Production Manager Susan Sutterby
Production Controller Claire Legg
Project Editor Katie Worrall

THE BRIDGEWATER BOOK COMPANY LTD
Art Director Terry Jeavons
Designer Glyn Bridgewater
Page layout Glyn Bridgewater
Managing Editor Anne Townley
Project Manager Fiona Corbridge
Picture Research Lynda Marshall
Three-dimensional models Mark Jamieson
Photography Ian Parsons
Illustrations Andrew Kulman

Printed and bound in Italy by Graphicom

British Library Cataloguing in
Publication data available

Library of Congress Cataloging
in Publication data available

ISBN 1 86204 197 0

The publishers wish to thank the following for the
use of pictures: Ancient Art and Architecture
Library: 6TL, 6BL; Bridgeman Art Library:
15BR; Hutchinson Library: 15TR; Image
Bank: 25B; Zefa: 21TR, 28R, 29L, 32L,
33, 37T, 37B, 41.

Special thanks go to: Nicola Pooley
and Annie Cryar, Lily Adams,
Robert Chappell, Natasha Gray,
Julia Holden, Natalie Jerome,
Caron Riley, Vincent Riley,
Jacob Swirsky *for help with*
photography.

Contents

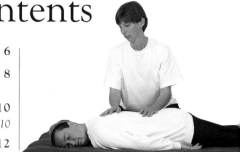

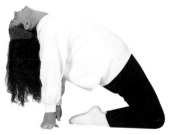

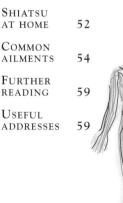

What is Shiatsu?

SHIATSU IS A JAPANESE FORM *of body work. It was developed from different disciplines of oriental medicine, including acupuncture and herbalism, as well as nutritional and exercise programs. Shiatsu, like many forms of massage, works to relax and invigorate the body. To this end, Shiatsu makes use of the body's natural energy.*

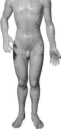

ABOVE: *An oriental statue showing the channels through which energy flows.*

Shiatsu originated in Japan as a holistic therapy for the treatment of mind, body, and spirit. When used correctly it is as useful for emotional pain as it is for physical problems.

The word "Shiatsu" comes from *shi*, meaning "finger" and *atsu*, meaning "pressure," although in reality Shiatsu may involve thumb, finger, elbow or even knee pressure. The

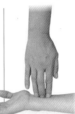

ABOVE: *Finger pressure taps into the body's own energy.*

quality of the pressure that is given is the most important feature that differentiates it from the many other forms of massage. To work with the body's energy the pressure must reach through the superficial layers of the body to its center. Sometimes this feels deeply relaxing and sometimes it can be quite painful.

Shiatsu is usually given on a futon, a Japanese mattress, with the giver and the recipient at floor level. The recipient remains clothed, which helps the practitioner contact the body's energy rather than the skin.

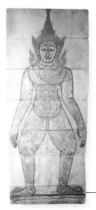

LEFT: *Using the traditional energy points, shown in this 19th-century diagram, Shiatsu treats symptoms and also their underlying causes.*

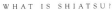
THE ENERGY OF LIFE

The energy of the body is called *ki* (pronounced "chee") in Japanese, *chi* or *qi* in Chinese and *prana* in Sanskrit. The energy refers to the quality of something which makes it alive – the energy to laugh and sing, or of flowers to grow through concrete. It is the energy of life.

THE BENEFITS OF SHIATSU

- Relaxes mind and body
- Restores and balances energy
- Eases tension and stiffness
- Improves breathing
- Improves circulation
- Heals
- Enhances well-being

BELOW: *In Shiatsu, the therapist may apply pressure to any of more than 600 traditional acupuncture points.*

The energy within the practitioner's body is balanced. This can be achieved by meditation before the Shiatsu session begins.

After consultation with the patient, specific problems can be addressed. The points on the body that are massaged are often located away from the problem area.

The practitioner aims to use both hands on the patient. Energy flows between the practitioner and patient in a closed circuit. In this case, one hand is just resting on the patient's body, while the other hand is working.

Shiatsu is given on a futon. This ensures the practitioner has a firm base to kneel on and can move around the patient easily.

The patient can feel their stress gradually dissolving away.

A short history

THE ORIGINS OF SHIATSU *can be traced back to Neolithic times – Neolithic people would have rubbed and pressed stiff and painful areas of their bodies much as we do. In the Far East a system of energy lines and points was developed over many centuries. Acupuncture as well as Shiatsu relies on this ancient oriental medical system, and the first stone needles used for this purpose are thought to be 9,000 years old.*

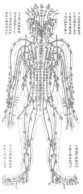

ABOVE: *Ancient charts show the energy lines of the body.*

Oriental medicine, and therefore Shiatsu, uses the philosophy of yin and yang. Yin is the quality of matter and substance, in other words the body, and yang is the quality of movement and thought – the energy. These qualities are further subdivided into the five elements: Earth, Metal, Water, Wood, and Fire. Each meridian, or pathway of energy in the body, is either yin or yang and associated with one of the five elements.

As Japan became more Westernized, Shiatsu was placed in a more anatomical and "physical" context. Most recently, the work of Masunaga synthesized traditional oriental medicine, Shiatsu, and physiology and psychology. This has made Shiatsu more accessible to Western students and is probably responsible for its emergence from the East.

Masunaga also developed a sophisticated form of diagnosis involving palpating the

THE NEI CHING

The earliest known oriental medical textbook, the *Nei Ching*, is said to have been written by Huang Ti, the legendary Yellow Emperor. It is first mentioned around 200 B.C.E., though it is almost certainly much older. The work is still a respected medical source in modern acupuncture.

abdomen – the *hara* – or the back. A description of this form of diagnosis is beyond the scope of this book, but it gives us an indication of the power of Shiatsu to heal by manipulating the energy, or ki, in the body.

STUDYING SHIATSU

Studying Shiatsu forms a spiral. At the first level it is enjoyable and healing for both the giver and recipient. The spiral continues, following the meridians or energy channels and taking the student on a journey of discovery. The energy of the meridians can affect the body, the mind, the emotions, and the spirit. Practitioners of Shiatsu are continually improving their technique to work more specifically on many levels.

RIGHT: **Shiatsu practitioners derive awareness and relaxation from the hara.**

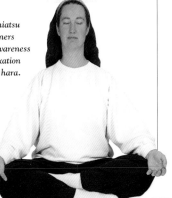

YIN AND YANG

Oriental medicine is based on the philosophy of yin and yang, the dual forces in the universe that are forever changing and which, in disease, go seriously out of balance, and the five phases or elements, which represent the ancient view of the changing seasons and the way human beings fit into them. If we don't live in harmony with the movements of nature, we become ill.

ABOVE: **The symbol for yin and yang shows them intertwined and interdependent.**

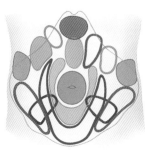

ABOVE: **The hara is the center of energy in the body.**

9

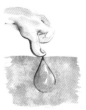

How does Shiatsu work?

ABOVE: *The flow of ki can be adjusted at specific "points" on the body. These points are like pools in a stream. Relaxed pressure is used.*

AT THE HEART OF SHIATSU is the aim of enabling ki to flow smoothly throughout the body meridians, but sometimes ki is blocked, and this can cause health problems. Shiatsu aims to relieve these blockages.

THE MERIDIANS

Meridians are the channels through which energy, or ki, flows in the body. Ki can be visualized much like water flowing: sometimes the river floods, sometimes it is dry. The meridians are like maps of rivers.

There are six pairs of meridians, which relate to different organs in the body.

SELF-SHIATSU ("Do-in")

One of the best ways to start Shiatsu is to explore the meridians on yourself. Press your body along the meridian lines and pay particular attention to any points which are sensitive. Discover the way that pressing the points can ease their

sensitivity and feel good. There may be a few surprises! Now try what you have learnt on someone else.

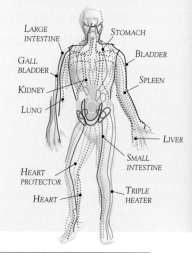

THE MERIDIANS ON THE FRONT OF THE BODY

LARGE INTESTINE

STOMACH

GALL BLADDER

BLADDER

KIDNEY

SPLEEN

LUNG

LIVER

SMALL INTESTINE

HEART PROTECTOR

HEART

TRIPLE HEATER

THE MERIDIANS AND THEIR ELEMENTS

- Lung and Large Intestine – *Metal*
- Stomach and Spleen – *Earth*
- Heart and Small Intestine – *Fire*
- Bladder and Kidney – *Water*
- Heart Protector and Triple Heater – *Fire*
- Gall Bladder and Liver – *Wood*

TOUCH

Human touch is one of the best healers of all. Using an instinctive touch with love and compassion can be spiritually healing. Think of the simple comfort you give when hugging a friend in need. This is the way to do Shiatsu.

SHIATSU SAFETY RULES

- Don't practise Shiatsu if another treatment is more appropriate.
- Don't work on open wounds, bruises, or varicose veins.
- Don't work too long or with too many specific points.
- Ask the recipient to let you know what feels uncomfortable or painful.
- Take care to avoid the points which are contraindicated (inadvisable) in pregnancy.
- The best safety rule of all is "When in doubt – don't."

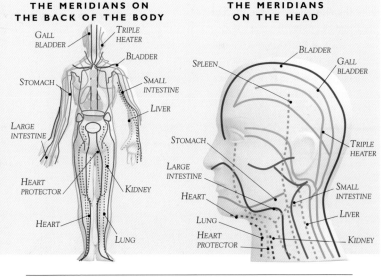

THE MERIDIANS ON THE BACK OF THE BODY

GALL BLADDER
TRIPLE HEATER
BLADDER
STOMACH
SMALL INTESTINE
LIVER
LARGE INTESTINE
HEART PROTECTOR
KIDNEY
HEART
LUNG

THE MERIDIANS ON THE HEAD

SPLEEN
BLADDER
GALL BLADDER
STOMACH
LARGE INTESTINE
HEART
LUNG
HEART PROTECTOR
TRIPLE HEATER
SMALL INTESTINE
LIVER
KIDNEY

Practising Shiatsu

IN SHIATSU THE GIVER *leans on the recipient using his or her body weight and moves along the meridians. There will be moments of stillness in the routine, and in this way Shiatsu differs from an ordinary massage.*

LEFT: *Lean forward to gently transfer your body weight to the recipient.*

BODY WEIGHT

When giving Shiatsu you should "relax" your weight – pushing or poking are painful for the recipient, whereas leaning is comfortable. On delicate parts such as the face, lean less, and on stronger areas like the buttocks, lean forward to put your body weight behind your hands or thumbs. Shiatsu is given at floor level, as it is easiest to lean into the recipient from a crawling position.

WALKING THE HANDS

Your hands or thumbs should walk or dance along the meridian lines. The rhythm should come instinctively from the quality of the recipient's energy – if they are tired it will become slower and if they are lively, faster. If this is difficult to ascertain, a natural walking pace is fine. Sometimes one hand will be still while the other hand walks away from it. Your technique will gradually improve with time.

RIGHT: *Walking the hands along the Heart Protector meridian in the arm. Match your pace to the recipient's energy level.*

BELOW: *A point may be held for a few seconds, and returned to several times.*

HOLDING POINTS

You will find that some areas of Shiatsu points need more attention than others. These areas and points can be held longer, but you should still continue to work on other areas. A particular point may be leant on for several seconds; however, it is better to return to a place several times than to lean on one spot for too long.

LISTEN WITH YOUR HANDS

Listen with your hands to what the recipient wants. Do whatever will make the recipient relax and feel comfortable.

USING YOUR THUMBS

The thumbs are used a lot in Shiatsu, as they fit well into most Shiatsu points and can be easily positioned. They should be relaxed – if there is any shaking or strain, they are too tense. Practise on your own leg. Relax your hand and your fingers will rest on the leg as your thumb moves along. The pressure should be firm but comfortable.

BELOW: *Practise your thumb technique on your own leg to begin with. Learn to gauge the pressure.*

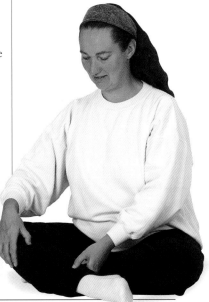

THE PRINCIPLES OF ZEN SHIATSU

Zen Shiatsu is a specific form of Shiatsu which is widely practised in the UK and US. The first exponent of this kind of Shiatsu, which tends to emphasize the relationship between psychological, spiritual, and emotional factors, and physical symptoms, was Shizuto Masunaga.

I RELAX

As the Shiatsu giver relaxes, this feeling is transmitted to the recipient. Relaxing also allows the giver to be more intuitive. Shiatsu should be relaxing for both people involved.

RIGHT: *It is essential for the Shiatsu giver to relax, or negative feelings will be felt by the recipient.*

2 USE TWO HANDS

Using two hands makes a circuit for the energy in the meridians. Try working on a foot with only one hand and then with two. It feels better and the effect is longer-lasting.

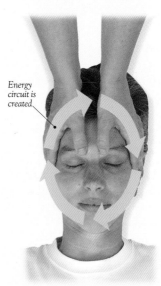

Energy circuit is created

ABOVE: *After practising the two-handed technique on other parts of the body, like the foot, it is possible to use it effectively in more sensitive areas.*

3 MERIDIAN CONTINUITY

Don't jump about. If you decide to work down the Water meridians on the front of the legs, finish that before moving on to another meridian.

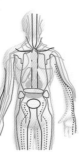

RIGHT:
Concentrate on one meridian at a time.

4 VERTICAL PRESSURE

When using an acupressure point or when working on the meridians it is essential to contact the person's energy. To do this the thumb has to be at a 90-degree angle to the point.

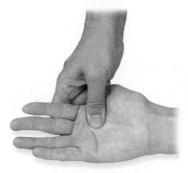

ABOVE: *The Heart Protector 8 point is found in the center of the palm. It is used to treat anxiety.*

5 THE HARA

The hara, or abdomen, is also the center of energy in the body. Martial artists, Japanese drummers and Shiatsu practitioners are all taught to work from this center. It helps them to be aware and relaxed. Learning comes from the center.

RIGHT: *Martial artists learn to channel energy from the hara into explosive movement.*

BUDDHAS

Buddhas are depicted with large abdomens to show how strong and full of energy their center is.

RIGHT:
In the Buddhist religion, buddhas are people who have achieved a state of perfect enlightenment.

A BASIC ROUTINE

Keep to a basic routine when practising Shiatsu until you are used to it. As you become more experienced you will become more intuitively aware of subtle changes in the recipient's energy.

PREPARATION

You will need:
- Quiet
- A warm, relaxing room
- A mattress or some blankets on the floor
- Loose, comfortable clothes
- A candle to create natural light and healing space

WITH THE RECIPIENT LYING FACE UP

1 Start with both hands gently connecting with the abdomen. Assess the general quality of the energy.

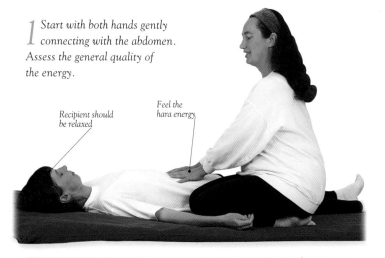

Recipient should be relaxed

Feel the hara energy

ASSESSING THE ENERGY

Listen with the hand to the energy of the body. Does it have plenty of energy? Is it tired? Is it humming like a tightly wired string? Use your imagination to picture the quality of the energy. Work with that quality during the Shiatsu session. At the end, check whether it has changed.

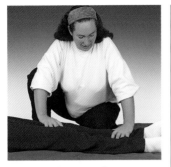

2 Crawl down one leg, using your body weight instinctively and leaning on areas that seem to require it.

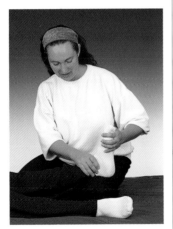

3 End with the foot. Strongly rotate the ankle and each toe. Help the energy reach the ends of the toes. Repeat for the other leg and foot.

THE NAILS

The energy of the meridians goes to all the nails of the fingers and toes. In Shiatsu it is important to draw the energy out to the nails. Squeeze the nails beside the "moons" and pull to the end of each finger and toe.

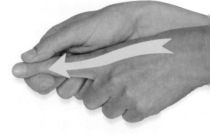

ABOVE: *Squeeze beside the nails, drawing down to the end of each finger.*

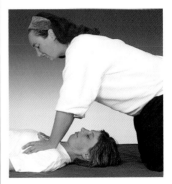

4 On the area above the lungs, use two hands and crawl or cat walk (see page 19).

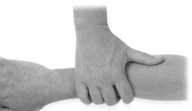

5 Smoothly crawl down the arm, leaning for longer on any areas that need attention.

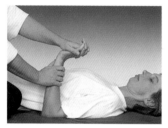

6 Firmly rotate the wrist and rotate each finger, bringing energy right to the ends of each meridian.

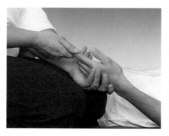

7 Repeat steps 5 and 6 for the other arm and hand.

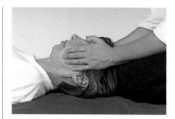

8 Move behind the head and work confidently over the face. Practise this on yourself first to find out what feels good.

THE FACE

Give firm Shiatsu to the face. Use one hand for support and follow the contours of the face across the forehead, around the eyes, down the nose, across the cheeks, and around the upper and lower jaw.

WITH THE RECIPIENT LYING FACE DOWN

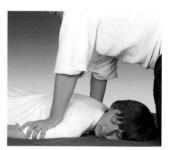

9 Crawl down the arms from above the head.

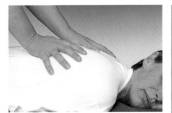

10 Move to the side and crawl or cat walk down the back. Avoid pressing directly on the bumps of the spine.

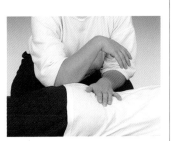

11 Lean into the buttocks – sometimes this is best done with the elbows.

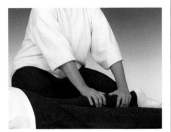

12 Crawl down one leg and then the other.

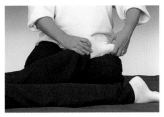

13 To finish, massage the feet.

CAT WALKING

Cat walking feels especially good. Cats have a special way of using their paws to knead the flesh (no claws!). Lean on to one palm and then the other. Use relaxed body weight, bringing more weight on to the firmer parts of the body.

ABOVE: *Bring out your feline qualities – ask your cat to show you how!*

ENHANCING YOUR ROUTINE

Add to the basic routine any appropriate techniques from the Elements section (see pages 24–45). During the routine, address extra points while working on the specific parts of the body.

Visiting a practitioner

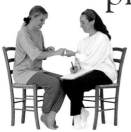

A SHIATSU SESSION WILL USUALLY take between 45 and 60 minutes. Before treatment starts, the practitioner will take a case history to establish which type of treatment will suit you best. After this comes your time to relax and enjoy the massage.

ABOVE: **Before treatment, a Shiatsu practitioner will want to take some medical details.**

You will be asked to lie down, probably on a Japanese mattress (futon) on the floor. You will remain clothed, so it is best to wear loose, comfortable clothes. A cotton jogging suit and socks are ideal. The practitioner will do a Shiatsu touch diagnosis, which means assessing the quality of your energy, probably via the hara, and will create a treatment specifically for you.

After Shiatsu people usually feel very relaxed. Sometimes they feel both relaxed and invigorated. To get the full benefit of the treatment, don't eat a big meal beforehand or rush off to an appointment afterward.

RIGHT: **The Shiatsu massage will be given to complement the energy levels you present at the time of treatment.**

Work takes place on the floor.

Some people feel great after a treatment, others can feel unwell for about 24 hours. This is because Shiatsu is aimed at stimulating the body to seek out and expel the deep-seated causes of health problems, and this can trigger a sort of "healing crisis" as toxins are released and ki is unblocked. Common symptoms include fatigue, headaches, flu-like symptoms and bowel changes. Try to relax until the symptoms pass, but call your therapist if they persist.

HOW TO FIND A PRACTITIONER

The national society (address at end of book) has lists of registered practitioners. Call the practitioner on the phone or arrange a meeting to see if you are suited. The best

recommendation is word of mouth from someone who has had Shiatsu.

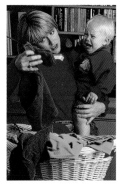

LEFT:
The tensions of domestic life can cause as much stress as the professional world.

WHICH PROBLEMS CAN SHIATSU HELP?

Shiatsu improves health generally by relieving stress, calming the nervous system, and stimulating the circulatory and immune systems. It is particularly effective for stress-related tension and illnesses, insomnia, back and joint pain, headaches, digestive upsets, sports injuries, menstrual pain, poor stamina, lack of libido, and as a preventive health measure.

WARNING

Always visit a physician or other health professional when symptoms are serious or persistent.

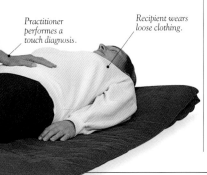

Practitioner performes a touch diagnosis.

Recipient wears loose clothing.

The five elements

THE MERIDIANS *are all divided into pairs which are yin and yang. The yang meridians are associated with energetic aspects of the body, such as movement and thought. The yin meridians are associated with more physical aspects, such as the organs and blood.*

ABOVE: *Yin and yang are used in Shiatsu at many levels.*

The five elements (Earth, Metal, Water, Wood and Fire) relate to different forms of ki. There is a yin and yang meridian associated with each element, except for Fire, which has two associated pairs of meridians. The elements each correspond to certain parts or functions of the body, as well as to certain emotions, and various phenomena which are thought to have a similar kind of energy.

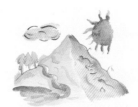

YIN AND YANG

Yin originally meant the shady side of the hill, while yang meant the sunny side. The sun moves round and what was shady becomes bright, but the hill remains the same.

THE SOUL

In traditional oriental thought the ethereal soul is that part of a person which continues after death, while the corporeal soul is that which dies with the body.

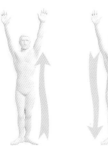

ABOVE: *Yin energy flows up the body in the meridians situated in the soft inner surfaces.*

ABOVE: *Yang energy flows down the body in the meridians situated nearer to the body surface.*

THE FIVE-ELEMENT ASSOCIATIONS

	Earth	Metal	Water	Wood	Fire
Yin organ	Spleen	Lung	Kidney	Liver	Heart and Heart Protector
Yang organ	Stomach	Large Intestine	Bladder	Gall Bladder	Small Intestine and Triple Heater
Body part	Connective tissue	Skin	Bones	Ligaments and tendons	Blood
Sense	Taste	Smell	Hearing	Sight	Speech
Voice	Singing	Weeping	Groaning	Shouting	Laughing
Emotion	Pensiveness	Grief	Fear	Anger	Joy
Spirit	Intellect	Corporeal soul	Will	Ethereal soul	Mind
Season	Late summer	Fall	Winter	Spring	Summer
Colour	Yellow	White	Blue/black	Green	Red

Earth

THE EARTH ELEMENT relates to how people look after themselves and how they care for others. Earth energy allows our caring to empower ourselves and those we care for, rather than fostering dependence.

EARTH RELATES TO

- Food and digestion
- Support and security
- Nurture and nourishment
- Center and grounding

Someone with harmonious Earth energy:

- Is grounded – a practical person who is not easily knocked off balance.
- Has a healthy appetite and a good relationship with food.
- Has good muscle tone with no sagging.
- Enjoys moderate exercise.
- Enjoys intellectual stimulation, such as studying, reading, and solving problems.
- Has a place which she calls her own.
- Has a good relationship with her mother.

FOOD

Good food is full of energy and is enjoyable. Fresh organic food contains more nutrients than junk food which is full of additives and preservatives. Brown rice has a life force, which means it can sprout.

UNHEALTHY FOODS FOR EARTH PEOPLE

- Refined sugars
- Mucus-producing food – dairy products, particularly cheese
- Too much raw food when the weather is cold
- Yeast

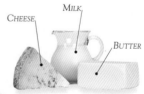

CHEESE   MILK   BUTTER

ABOVE: **When Earth energy is low, avoid dairy products.**

LEFT: **An Earth child gets on well with her mother.**

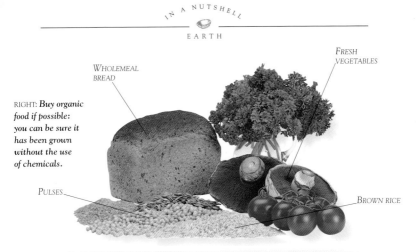

WHOLEMEAL
BREAD

FRESH
VEGETABLES

RIGHT: **Buy organic
food if possible:
you can be sure it
has been grown
without the use
of chemicals.**

PULSES

BROWN RICE

HOW EARTH ENERGY GETS OUT OF BALANCE

Bad habits with food

- Irregular eating weakens the Earth. Regular meals – especially breakfast – help.
- Eating on the run, or whilst reading, upsets digestion.

Lack of exercise

When the muscles lose tone, the body begins to sag internally and externally. Exercise such as walking, gardening and dancing all benefit the connective tissue.

Worry

Worry ties the brain in knots and tangles Earth energy. Shiatsu calms troubled thoughts.

Insecurity

Moving house, traveling, and staying in other people's houses all disturb the Earth energy.

Caring

Earth energy is easily upset if the balance between caring for others and for oneself is out of adjustment. This is a problem in many professions, such as nursing and social work.

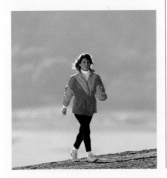

LEFT: **The simplest of exercises,
such as walking, can help
balance Earth energy.**

STOMACH AND SPLEEN MERIDIANS

The element Earth is associated with the Stomach and Spleen meridians, which influence the whole of the front of the body.

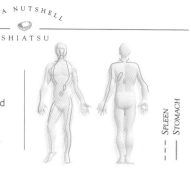

--- *SPLEEN*
——— *STOMACH*

TO CHANNEL EARTH ENERGY

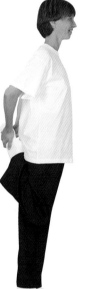

1 Stand with both feet under the shoulders and without moving the hips much. Lift one leg and grip the foot with your hand. Stretch.

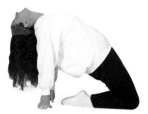

2 Kneel up with the hips between the heels. Gently lift the hips until a stretch is felt on the front of the legs. Relax the head back.

3 Something to aim for! Start as you did for Step 2. With the hips between the heels, lie back onto the elbows, shoulders, and – if it is easy – to the floor. Don't strain to achieve this.

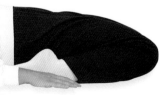

SHIATSU FOR EARTH ENERGY

☞ Wobbling the body relaxes all the connective tissue as well as preventing worry. (Try to worry while being wobbled!) To wobble somebody, make bony contact, for example with the hips, and then wobble the muscles. (To wobble a jelly we hold the plate.)

☞ Give Shiatsu down the front of the legs on the Stomach and Spleen meridians. Pay special attention to the knees. End by giving the feet a strong massage.

☞ Facial massage is good for Earth energy, particularly on the forehead and cheeks. Work from the hairline down to the neck.

☞ Gentle massage of the abdomen, or hara, is very centering. This can be done either with two hands or with one on the lower back and one on the hara.

BELOW: *Wobbling relaxes muscles and ligaments. Lack of muscle tone is a feature of unbalanced Earth energy.*

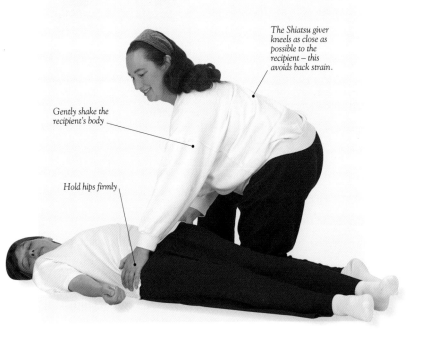

The Shiatsu giver kneels as close as possible to the recipient – this avoids back strain.

Gently shake the recipient's body

Hold hips firmly

Metal

THE METAL ELEMENT *relates to how people see themselves; how they set up boundaries between themselves and the rest of the world. This is reflected in breathing: whether air flows easily from the world into the body and out again, or whether there is a permanent struggle between what is taken and what is given back.*

METAL RELATES TO

- Breathing in and breathing out
- Taking in and letting go
- Clarity and understanding
- Borders and boundaries

RIGHT:
The clear skin of someone with balanced Metal energy.

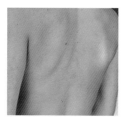

BREATHING

Breathing connects humans to the energy of the universe. When breathing in, we take in the energy of heaven – cosmic energy. This gives us life. Many spiritual practices use breathing – "the breath" – to connect to that which is divine.

Someone with harmonious Metal energy:

- Copes with letting go of the past and making space to step into the future.
- Creates space in his life by throwing out old things.
- Has no problems with breathing, and after strenuous exercise the breath quickly returns to normal.
- Has good skin.
- Has a clear sense of self and knows his own boundaries.
- Has clarity of thought and is capable of organized thinking.
- Has an ability to create networks socially and at work.
- Has a good relationship with his father.

ABOVE: *Even after strenuous exercise, breathing soon returns to normal if you have good Metal energy.*

HOW METAL ENERGY GETS OUT OF BALANCE

Not letting go of emotional pain

The grieving process is a healthy one which makes room for new experiences. Although grieving is painful, avoiding it will damage Metal energy. Rituals and remembering sad events help grieving.

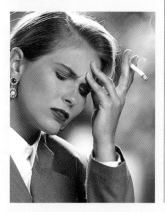

Not eliminating

Problems with the bowels can upset Metal energy. Regular bowels mean different things to different people. There is no right rhythm except the one that is comfortable.

Smoking

Smoking causes severe damage to Metal energy as it affects breathing, represses emotional pain, and causes damage to the body. (*See* Common Ailments section, page 54.)

Loneliness

When someone spends more time alone than is desired, it can upset Metal energy. Being content and alone is one thing, but loneliness hurts.

LEFT: *The health risks of smoking are well known. It also contracts Metal energy.*

FIBER

Healthy bowels need a diet that includes enough unprocessed vegetable food, or fiber. To get enough fiber, a healthy diet should contain at least five portions of fresh fruit or vegetables (not including potatoes) a day.

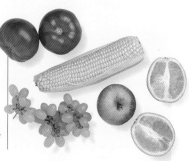

RIGHT: *You should find it easy to eat at least five portions of fresh fruit and vegetables daily.*

LUNG AND LARGE INTESTINE MERIDIANS

The element Metal is associated with the Lung and Large Intestine meridians, which influence the outside of the body – the physical boundary, or the skin.

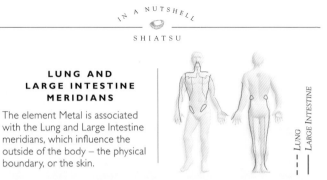

- - - LUNG
—— LARGE INTESTINE

TO CHANNEL METAL ENERGY

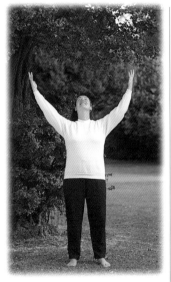

1 Breathe deeply and expand the chest. While breathing in, open and lift the arms, and while breathing out, slowly lower the arms. This is best done outside under a leafy tree.

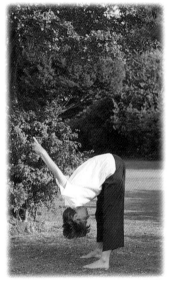

2 Link the thumbs behind the back, and breathe in. While breathing out, lean forward. Hang down and lift the arms toward the sky. Breathe slowly. Return slowly to upright position.

SHIATSU FOR METAL ENERGY

☞ Work with the recipient's breathing. Place the palms on the lungs in the upper chest, and ask the recipient to breathe in. As she breathes out, lean some weight on to the lungs to help exhalation. This can also be done diagonally with one hand on the upper chest and one on the ribs.

☞ Give Shiatsu to the Lung and Large Intestine meridians on the arms. Keep one hand on the lungs and continue to work with the breath.

☞ Shiatsu on the abdomen is useful for the large intestine – work deeply around the abdomen in a clockwise direction. It is also good to rotate the hips.

☞ Shiatsu on the buttocks is great for Metal energy. Try to encourage the recipient to sigh or breathe out while firmly leaning into the buttocks.

BELOW: *Working on the buttocks will restore metal energy. Ensure that the recipient breathes in tune with you as you work.*

Use your elbow to lean into the buttocks

Breathes out as you lean

MODELING

When working with the breath, it is important that the giver also breathes out as the recipient breathes out. This reciprocal principle can work for any technique. If you are trying to relax the recipient's shoulder, you need to relax your own shoulders.

Water

THE WATER ELEMENT *relates to a person's constitution, which is passed down from the parents and is reflected in bones, hair, posture, and memory. A person with a good constitution has plenty of energy and drive to fulfill ambitions.*

WATER RELATES TO

- Courage and bravery
- Drive and impetus
- Past and future
- Balance and moderation

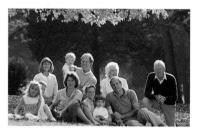

ABOVE: *Maintaining close family ties is important to the person with well-balanced Water energy.*

Someone with harmonious Water energy:

- Has realistic goals and ambitions, and the energy to achieve them.
- Has a good relationship with family, extended family, and ancestors.
- Takes an occasional alcoholic drink, coffee or tea – but nothing in excess.
- Has a good constitution, good health, and a reliable memory.
- Needs some excitement and danger, but will limit herself to appropriate risk-taking.
- Has a strong back, and a healthy posture.

ENERGY

The energy we get from our parents at conception – ancestral energy – is stored with Water energy. This is gradually used up through our life. Our energy is expended more quickly if we live in the fast lane.

BELOW: *Ancestral energy is at a maximum level when we are babies.*

HOW WATER ENERGY GETS OUT OF BALANCE

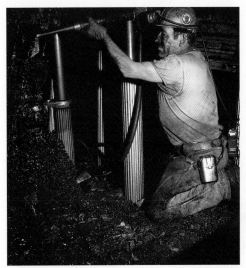

LEFT: *People whose work is physically demanding are especially likely to run down their Water energy.*

Overwork
☞ Continual work, either stressful mental activity or hard physical labor, can deplete Water energy. (Especially if the candle is being burnt at both ends!)

☞ When one needs to work for long hours it is important to schedule in some rest.

Cold
☞ Cold weather, cold environments, and not wearing enough clothes particularly around the lower back, will weaken Water energy.

Traumas
☞ Frightening or shocking experiences such as physical accidents or emotional hurts can damage Water energy. People need time, with good rest, to recover from such experiences.

Abuse of stimulants
☞ Using either legal drugs, such as coffee, or illegal drugs to keep going will severely damage Water energy and will deplete ancestral energy. Moderation in all things is the key to harmony.

☞ The occasional coffee does no harm to a healthy person – 4, 5, or 6 cups a day is excessive.

KIDNEY AND BLADDER MERIDIANS

The element Water is associated with the Bladder and Kidney meridians which hold up the back.

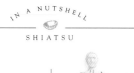

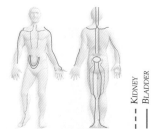

--- *Kidney*
— *Bladder*

TO CHANNEL WATER ENERGY

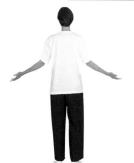

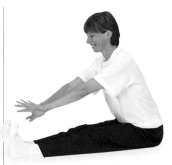

1 Imagine breathing from the top of your head and taking the breath down through your spine, all the way to your tailbone. Imagine the breath bringing silver light, healing, and space around each bone.

2 Sit on the floor with the legs outstretched. Look forward and stretch forward to touch the toes. Again release the spine and try to relax the backs of the legs.

POSTURE

Good posture means being able to stand up straight with the head balanced on the neck and spine. The chin is tucked in so the neck is not compressed.

The hips are relaxed. The bones of the back are held in place by posture, not muscles.

34

SHIATSU FOR WATER ENERGY

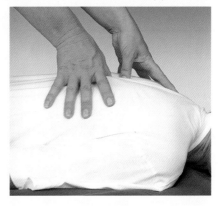

Apply firm pressure

Move the bones against each other

☞ Shiatsu for Water energy has to connect to the bones. This needs a deep and firm pressure. Try it on yourself first. Try holding the bones of the fingers and moving them against each other. Small movements can bring Water energy into the bones.

ABOVE: **The bones reflect constitutional elements that are inherited.**

RIGHT: **Cat walking down the spine (see page 19). Take special care when working on someone's back.**

☞ Shiatsu can benefit the back. A beginner should get plenty of feedback from the recipient. Start with cat walking down the back of each of the knobbly bits of the spine, taking care not to apply pressure to the knobs themselves.

☞ Do exercise 1 (on the facing page) together. The Shiatsu giver needs to breathe down her own spine as well as breathing down the recipient's spine. This is subtle work but can be very powerful.

ARTHRITIS

Shiatsu is good for arthritis, but you should never work on the joints when they are hot or inflamed. Otherwise, the most important thing is to keep the joints moving.

Deep, slow movements which bring energy and nutrition into the joint can eventually bring a lot of movement back into joints that have "seized up" or become stiff.

Wood

THE WOOD ELEMENT *relates to how a person responds to the world. Wood energy enables people to be free spirits who live creatively, or to have great plans and use the world around them for their own goals.*

WOOD RELATES TO

- Freedom and flexibility
- Creativity and control
- Expression and effectiveness
- Detoxification and decision-making

Someone with harmonious Wood energy:

- Is a creative person who brings creativity into their life.
- Has a flexible body and is able to bend and stretch.
- Has a flexible mind which is not prejudiced and is always open to new ideas.
- Is confident at making decisions and functions well in a crisis.

- Has a good liver, so is able to digest rich food and the occasional alcoholic drink.

LEFT: *A rich diet does not cause indigestion in a strong Wood personality.*

THE LIVER

The liver is like a factory processing plant for the body. It processes fats, alcohol, excess proteins, and toxins.

RIGHT:
Flexibility is a key characteristic of people with good Wood energy.

HOW WOOD ENERGY GETS OUT OF BALANCE

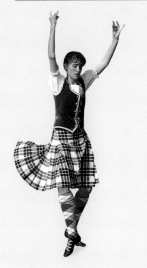

ABOVE: *Dancing is fun, good exercise, and helps to balance Wood energy.*

Dancing, tennis, going to the gym, in fact, any form of exercise which includes fun is good for Wood energy.

Repression of strong emotions

Everyone has feelings and everyone gets annoyed – all of which is healthy. When people don't admit these feelings, maybe not even to themselves, then problems can occur.

Stress

Stressful situations, where decisions are continually being made, can easily upset Wood energy. Delegation and support are essential at these times.

Control

Over-control of the body or of the environment will upset the free nature of Wood energy.

Over-indulgence

Drinking too much alcohol or eating fatty foods (or both) regularly will weaken Wood energy.

Not enough movement

Keeping the body in a rigid posture, or simply lack of exercise, can damage Wood energy and lead to stiffness.

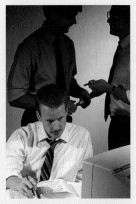

ABOVE: *Try not to let workplace stress get the better of you. Delegate as much as possible.*

LIVER AND GALL BLADDER MERIDIANS

The element Wood is associated with the Liver and Gall Bladder meridians. These are situated on the sides of the body and are important for bending and twisting.

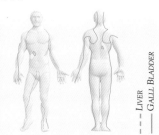

--- LIVER
—— GALLL BLADDER

TO CHANNEL WOOD ENERGY

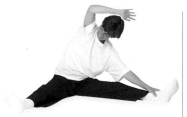

1 Sit on the floor with your legs spread wide apart. Reach down to your left foot, looking at your right foot. Stretch the sides of your legs and the sides of your body. Repeat on the other side.

2 Stand up with your feet apart. Let your arms start swinging from side to side. Feel the air on your arms. Keep swinging for a few minutes.

WOOD ENERGY

When Wood energy is upset it tends to become "stagnant" and not flow round the body freely. It becomes stagnant mainly at the joints, particularly the large joints, which become stiff. To free Wood energy, the body needs to stretch and be stretched.

LEFT: *Simple stretching exercises prevent the joints from becoming stiff.*

SHIATSU FOR WOOD ENERGY

☞ The ball-and-socket joints of the hips and shoulders benefit from being rotated. Lift the recipient's leg or arm and support the shoulder or hip. The recipient needs to feel the rotation. Try to make it smooth.

☞ Wood energy flows when it is stretched. During the rotations, see if you can find a place at which the joint sticks a bit. This is the place to stretch. Gently pull the limb. Then hold the stretch for a few moments. Get feedback from the recipient. It should feel good, not painful.

☞ Give Shiatsu to the Wood meridians (the Liver and Gall Bladder) on the inside and outside of the legs.

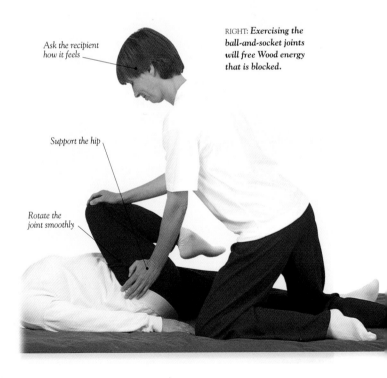

RIGHT: *Exercising the ball-and-socket joints will free Wood energy that is blocked.*

Ask the recipient how it feels

Support the hip

Rotate the joint smoothly

Fire

THE FIRE ELEMENT *has two strands. The Fire which is associated with people's relationship with themselves and the universe is called Spirit Fire. The Fire concerned with relationships to other people is called Human Fire.*

**SPIRIT FIRE
RELATES TO**

☞ Self and not self
☞ Mind and spirit
☞ Joy and contentment

Someone with harmonious Spirit Fire energy:

☞ Is at peace with herself and the universe.

☞ Is mentally well balanced and emotionally stable.

☞ Has a sense of joy in her life and laughs easily when it is appropriate.

☞ Has a sense of awe at the marvels of the universe. She may enjoy gazing at a beautiful sunset, or may have a strong religious conviction.

☞ Is calm when it is needed.

☞ May be intuitive or seem to have a sixth sense.

☞ Assimilates what she needs to be herself, either physically via the small intestine, or emotionally, to keep an even keel.

LEFT: *Meditation strengthens Spirit Fire energy, and reinforces a sense of purpose in life.*

HUMAN FIRE
RELATES TO

- Self and others
- Intimacy and closeness
- Protection and survival

**Someone with harmonious
Human Fire energy:**

- Is good company.
- Isn't easily embarrassed.
- Is relaxed in large
groups and in small,
intimate relationships.
- Feels comfortable giving
gifts and attention, and
receiving the same.
- Has a clear sense of
his own personal space
and adapts it to meet
different situations.

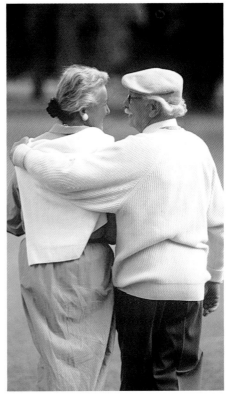

RIGHT: *Good Human Fire
energy is the key to long-lasting
relationships, where people are
happy to show their feelings.*

PERSONAL SPACE

Everyone has a personal space which adapts to the environment. When we are alone in our own home, our personal space may fill that home. As we go out on the street it shrinks considerably. If we were to get on a crowded bus, our personal space would then pull in close. If someone undesirable stands too near to us it becomes more protected. If a friend is on the bus with us, together we make a common, private, and personal space.

HOW FIRE ENERGY
GETS OUT OF BALANCE

RIGHT:
The close family bonds made in childhood are important for forging strong Fire energy as an adult.

Communication
☞ When there are problems communicating with friends or family, this will easily disturb Fire energy.

☞ Counseling courses and confidence-building may help.

Childhood relationships
☞ Fire energy is about the emotional body. This is formed in childhood and, as everyone knows, how we are brought up has a profound effect on the adult. If children don't receive enough love, security, or compassion as they are learning about their emotional selves, Fire energy will be upset.

☞ It will help if adults learn to love "the child within."

Emotional trauma
☞ All emotional traumas affect the body's energy in many ways. But as a first layer of protection there is Fire energy.

☞ Too many emotional traumas weaken Fire energy.

Lack of personal space
☞ Living in a close community can be fun, but if there is no time to be oneself then Fire energy gets upset.

☞ Meditation, quiet times, or prayer all benefit Fire energy.

LEFT:
Focus on a candle while you meditate, to improve concentration.

HEART AND SMALL INTESTINE MERIDIANS

The element Fire is associated with Heart and Small Intestine meridians. These connect with our inner self.

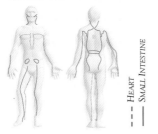

- - - HEART
—— SMALL INTESTINE

HEART PROTECTOR AND TRIPLE HEATER

Heart Protector and Triple Heater meridians influence the surface of the body and our personal space, temperature control, and the flow of energy in the body.

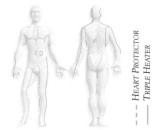

- - - HEART PROTECTOR
—— TRIPLE HEATER

THE TRIPLE HEATER

☞ The Upper Heater is the area of the heart and lungs, and is where we connect to the energy of heaven via the breath and our spirit.

☞ The Middle Heater is the area of the stomach and digestion, and is where we connect to the energy of the earth by taking in food and nourishment.

☞ The Lower Heater is the area of the hara and genitals; this is where we store energy for ourselves and for the next generation. It is also the area of the bladder and intestines.

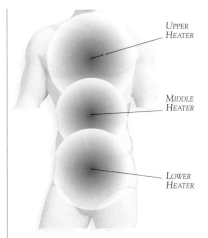

UPPER HEATER

MIDDLE HEATER

LOWER HEATER

ABOVE: *The meridians relate to different organs, but some, such as the Triple Heater, do not have an equivalent organ.*

43

TO CHANNEL FIRE ENERGY

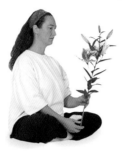

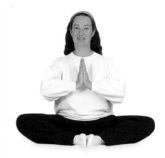

1 Meditation – sit with an object of beauty, such as a candle, flower, or crystal. With your eyes slightly out of focus, keep your attention on the object and be aware of the rhythm of your breath. Sit for a few minutes to begin with and build up to longer periods.

2 Sit with your heels together and pulled up to your body. Put your hands into a prayer position, with space under your armpits. Lean forward and breathe into the heart area. This is a classic "contemplating the navel" position! It works well to balance Fire energy.

3 Sit in a cross-legged position. Start in whatever position is comfortable for you. If you can get one foot on the other (half or full-lotus yoga posture) do so, otherwise just cross your legs. Then with the arms crossed, stretch over the knees and lean forward. Breathe into the heart area.

SHIATSU FOR FIRE ENERGY

☞ Shiatsu for the Fire meridians needs to be calm. Give light Shiatsu to the chest and arms with the intention of letting Fire glow but not blaze up.

☞ Balance the relationship between the mind, heart, and body. Do this by lightly resting one hand on the hara and the other on the heart area. Wait until they feel similar. Do the same for the heart and head.

☞ Shoulders. Rotate the arm, with the recipient lying on her back. Then slide one hand under the shoulder and hold the shoulder blade. Hold the top of the shoulder with the other hand. With both hands together, smoothly circle the shoulder.

☞ Sometimes working on Fire meridians can leave people feeling light-headed. If this happens, end the session by holding the heels.

BELOW: *Harmonizing mind, heart, and body by tuning in to the heart – the body's energy center.*

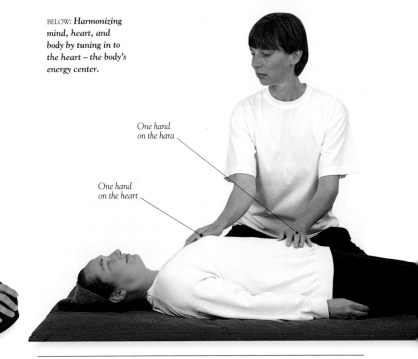

One hand on the hara

One hand on the heart

Shiatsu points

THE POINTS USED in Shiatsu are the classical acupuncture points, or Tsubo. They are the places where ki accumulates and therefore where it can most easily be accessed and manipulated. Each one is numbered according to its position on the meridian.

THE STOMACH AND SPLEEN MERIDIANS

- - - SPLEEN
—— STOMACH

STOMACH 8
Corner of the Head
☞ On the forehead at the corner of the hairline.
☞ It calms and clears the head, and is good for frontal headaches caused by worry.

STOMACH 36
Leg Three Mile
☞ A hand-width below the kneecap on the outside of the shin bone.
☞ A general tonic point which strengthens digestion and blood.

☞ Traditionally, soldiers would massage this point when they needed to walk an extra three miles.
☞ It can be used for stomach ache, constipation, and fatigue.

SPLEEN 6
Three Yin
Contraindicated in pregnancy.
☞ A hand-width above the inside ankle bone. Improves the yin and muscle tone.
☞ Regulates menstruation and digestion.

SPLEEN 9
Yin Mound Spring
☞ At the bottom of the bony bump on the inside of the knee.
☞ This point removes damp and so is good for diarrhea, cystitis, and water retention.

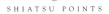
LUNG AND LARGE INTESTINE MERIDIANS

When the breath is shallow the Lung is indicated. If there is difficulty breathing, the Large Intestine is more appropriate.

- - - LUNG
——— LARGE INTESTINE

LUNG 1
Central Meeting
☞ In the hollow below the end of the collarbone. A great point for gradually opening the chest.
☞ For the lungs and for low vitality.
☞ Also for coughs, asthma, and any congestion in the chest.

LUNG 9 *Great Abyss*
☞ In the wrist crease below the thumb.
☞ An accessible point with a strong beneficial action on the lungs.
☞ It is good when giving up smoking, as it benefits the lungs and gives the hands something to do.
☞ Also for coughs and asthma.

LARGE INTESTINE 4
Great Eliminator
Contraindicated in pregnancy.
☞ At the height of the web between the thumb and forefinger.
☞ Eliminates pain anywhere in the body.
☞ Also good for constipation.
☞ Use during labor.

LARGE INTESTINE 20
Welcome Fragrance
☞ Next to the nostrils in a slight depression.
☞ Rub down the sides of the nose until there is a natural hollow.
☞ Clears the head.
☞ For sinusitis and hay fever.

DAMP

In oriental medicine damp means phlegm, mucus, or excess water.

HEART AND SMALL INTESTINE MERIDIANS

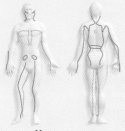

--- HEART
— SMALL INTESTINE

HEART 7
Gate of God
☞ In the wrist crease below the little finger.
☞ Calms the mind and the heart.
☞ For anxiety, hysteria, and insomnia.

HEART 9 *Lesser Yin Rushing*
☞ At the inside corner of the little fingernail.
☞ Use for the energy of the heart.
☞ Good for palpitations and chest pain.

SMALL INTESTINE 3
Back Stream
☞ A third of the way along the outside of a loose fist.
☞ A point for relaxing muscles and tendons in the back, shoulders, and neck. Use for neckache, stiff shoulder, and back pain.

SMALL INTESTINE 10
Arm Transporting
☞ On the back of the shoulder, below the end spine of the shoulder.
☞ This point can be painful with stiff muscles and congested energy.
☞ Use to release the energy of the neck and shoulders.
☞ Also for releasing the bones in the head, especially ears.

SMALL INTESTINE 19
Palace of Hearing
☞ Next to the ear in a little hollow which appears when the jaw is relaxed.
☞ Good for the ears – tinnitus, deafness, and earache.

THE KIDNEY AND BLADDER MERIDIANS

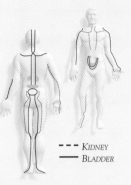

- - - KIDNEY
—— BLADDER

KIDNEY 1
Bubbling Spring
- In the center of the foot, a third of the way down from the toes.
- A lovely point which gives energy to the whole body and calms the mind. For headaches, fatigue, anxiety, and insomnia.

KIDNEY 3
Greater Stream
- Between the Achilles tendon and the inside ankle bone.
- Strengthens the whole body, particularly the uterus.
- For absence of periods and heavy periods, and for backache.

KIDNEY 7
Returning Current
- Above Kidney 3.
- Strengthens the kidneys directly and is good for water retention.
- Also for diarrhea, cystitis, and night sweats.

BLADDER 2
Collecting Bamboo
- At the inside corner of the eyebrows.
- A great point for hay fever and sinusitis.
- Good for headaches, especially those caused by overwork.

BLADDER 23
Kidney Yu Point

- To find them on oneself, hold the waist with the hand resting on the hips, thumbs forward. The fingertips will rest either side of the spine.
- A tonic for the whole body.
- For all forms of tiredness, fatigue, and for lower backache.

HEART PROTECTOR AND
TRIPLE HEATER MERIDIANS

The Heart Protector meridian – sometimes called the Pericardium – affects the pumping of the heart organ more than the Heart meridian, which relates to mental and spiritual aspects of a person.

--- HEART PROTECTOR
—— TRIPLE HEATER

HEART PROTECTOR 8
Palace of Anxiety
☞ Found in the center of the palm, where the third fingertip rests in a loosely clenched fist.
☞ Calms the mind.
☞ The lotus chakra and stigmata point – a sacred point.
☞ A great point for all forms of anxiety.

HEART PROTECTOR 6
Inner Gate
☞ Three finger-widths above the wrist crease in the center of the inner arm.
☞ For nausea, especially caused by emotion or motion.
☞ Morning sickness and travel sickness.
☞ Also for palpitations, insomnia, and chest pain.

TRIPLE HEATER 5
Outer Gate
☞ The opposite side of the arm to Heart Protector 6.
☞ It also has a similar action.
☞ For nausea.

TRIPLE HEATER 23
Silk Bamboo Hole
☞ At the outside end of the eyebrow where the eyebrow leaves the bone.
☞ A useful point for all problems of the head.
☞ For headache, toothache, and earache.

LIVER AND GALL BLADDER MERIDIANS

STAGNATION

Liver and Gall Bladder energy often gets congested or stagnant, which causes aches, stiffness, or pain. The points have strong actions to move blocked energy.

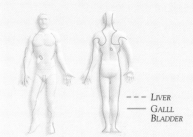

--- *Liver*
— *Gall Bladder*

GALL BLADDER 20
Wind Pond
- At the end of the tendons which attach to the base of the head – the occiput.
- An excellent point for headaches.
- For migraine, one-sided, and occipital headaches.

GALL BLADDER 21
Shoulder Well
Contraindicated in pregnancy
- Half-way along the top of the shoulder.
- This point is often congested and can be sore.
- Working the point will remove congestion and send energy down.
- Use to free the head, neck, and shoulder.
- Also for labor.

LIVER 3
Great Surge
- At the height of the web between the first and second toes.
- A sedative point for pain.
- Especially good for migraine and one-sided headaches, irregular and painful periods, and muscle cramps and spasms.

LIVER 14
Gate of Hope
- Below the nipple, in the 6th intercostal (the bra line).
- This point opens the chest and is good for heartburn, indigestion, and pain in the chest.
- Also useful for depression.

Shiatsu at home

SHIATSU CAN BE DONE AT HOME – *addressing points on your own body or that of someone else. When you have found the location of the point on the body, try pressing it. Remember to lean into the point and to go in at 90 degrees. It helps to imagine breathing out through the thumb into the point. Hold the point for a few seconds, repeat several times.*

ABOVE: *Try pressing the Liver 3 point to conquer a migraine.*

Don't press points for too long. It is best to include the points in a self-Shiatsu routine. In a full Shiatsu massage the points will be chosen after a diagnosis of the whole person. It is even better to get a friend to lean on the points for you during a Shiatsu session.

When giving Shiatsu at home, be sure you follow the basic guidelines on p.11.

Find a quiet space where you won't be interrupted.

Adopt a comfortable position. Choose a chair that is the correct height for you.

RIGHT: *Self-Shiatsu, or "Do-in," is useful for immediate relief of minor ailments.*

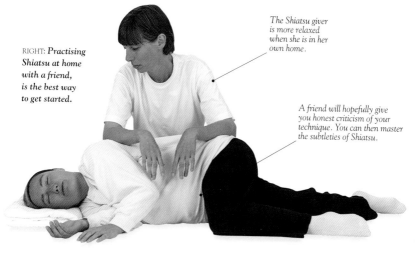

RIGHT: *Practising Shiatsu at home with a friend, is the best way to get started.*

The Shiatsu giver is more relaxed when she is in her own home.

A friend will hopefully give you honest criticism of your technique. You can then master the subtleties of Shiatsu.

STRETCHING

In the morning, a stretch and a yawn wakes the whole body. Stretches help to release the muscles and the joints, and move blocked energy. Stretches can be done alone, using particular poses, or any position that feels good. Stretches are also an integral part of Shiatsu where hips, shoulders, fingers, and toes are generally stretched.

Whether stretching by oneself or as part of a Shiatsu routine with a partner, remember to breathe out while moving into a stretch position. In Shiatsu, the giver should harmonize their

outward breath with the recipient's outward breath. Breathing out allows the diaphragm to relax, which in turn encourages all the internal organs to relax. Hold the stretch position while breathing in. Stretch further with each outward breath. Stretch only as far as is comfortable, because pain will bring tension.

WARNING

Always listen to your body, and to the feedback from the person you are treating. Stop if something feels uncomfortable.

Common ailments

ALTHOUGH REGULAR SHIATSU *massage will ensure that your body systems are working at an optimal level, the points which are particularly helpful to specific conditions are described below.*

CHEST PAIN AND PALPITATIONS

☞ Gentle Shiatsu on the Fire meridians, being careful to include all the fingers and toes. Hold the heart area with one hand and the abdomen with the other.

- Heart 7 *(p.48)*
- Heart 9 *(p.48)*
- Heart Protector 6 *(p.50)*

ASTHMA

☞ Don't work during an attack. Otherwise give regular Shiatsu to open the chest and on the Metal and Water meridians. Aim to relax the breath.

- Lung 1 *(p.47)*
- Lung 9 *(p.47)*
- Kidney 1 *(p.49)*

COUGHS

☞ Shiatsu to open the chest, and on the Metal and Wood meridians.

☞ Using the points for first aid is effective.

- Lung 1 *(p.47)*
- Lung 9 *(p.47)*

HAY FEVER

☞ With hay fever it is always best to start working with self-Shiatsu in February.

☞ Regular, firm Shiatsu to Earth, Water, and Metal meridians.

- Large Intestine 20 *(p.47)*
- Bladder 2 *(p.49)*
- Stomach 8 *(p.46)*

SINUSITIS

☞ Give plenty of Shiatsu to the face, and down the Earth and Metal meridians. Give strong pressure down the sides of the nose. Finish at the feet and rotate the toes.

- Large Intestine 20 *(p.47)*
- Stomach 8 *(p.46)*
- Bladder 2 *(p.49)*

EAR PROBLEMS

☞ Give Shiatsu on the face and ears.

☞ Holding the palms over the ears can benefit them.

☞ Also work the feet and pay attention to the Water meridians.

- Small Intestine 19 *(p.48)*
- Small Intestine 10 *(p.48)*
- Triple Heater 23 *(p.50)*
- Kidney 1 *(p.49)*

TINNITUS

☞ General Shiatsu to relax and restore the energy as tinnitus is often a sign of low energy.

- Small Intestine 19 *(p.48)*
- Kidney 1 *(p.49)*

EYE PROBLEMS

☞ Give Shiatsu on the face and round the eyes.

☞ Holding the palms over the eyes can give good results if done regularly.

- Gall Bladder 20 *(p.51)*
- Bladder 2 *(p.49)*
- Triple Heater 23 *(p.50)*

TOOTHACHE

☞ Shiatsu is useful for relaxation.

☞ Use the points specifically for the toothache.

- Large Intestine 4 *(p.47)*
- Small Intestine 19 *(p.48)*
- Triple Heater 23 *(p.50)*

CYSTITIS

☞ Give regular Shiatsu to the Earth and Water meridians, especially on the legs and the feet.

☞ Gentle holding of the abdomen with one hand, with the other on the sacrum, can help.

- Spleen 9 *(p.46)*
- Kidney 1 *(p.49)*
- Kidney 7 *(p.49)*

CONSTIPATION

☞ Working round the abdomen in a clockwise direction often helps.

☞ Firm Shiatsu for Metal, Wood, and Earth meridians.

☞ Hip rotations can help.

- Large Intestine 4 *(p.47)*
- Stomach 36 *(p.46)*
- Gall Bladder 21 *(p.51)*

DIARRHEA

☞ Gentle Shiatsu on the legs, especially the Earth and Water meridians.

- Spleen 9 *(p.46)*
- Kidney 7 *(p.49)*
- and if the diarrhea alternates with constipation use Large Intestine 4 *(p.47)*

STOMACH ACHE

☞ Gentle Shiatsu on the abdomen can help, but make sure a professional diagnosis is made first.

☞ Give Shiatsu on the Earth meridians on legs and feet.

- Stomach 36 (p.46)
- Spleen 6 (p.46)
- Heart Protector 6 (p.50)

HEARTBURN
AND INDIGESTION

☞ Work on the abdomen in a clockwise direction.

☞ Give Shiatsu to the Fire and Wood meridians.

- Liver 14 (p.51)
- Heart Protector 8 (p.50)

ANXIETY

☞ Shiatsu, like all massage, is particularly good for stress and anxiety. Use gentle and continuous Shiatsu, especially on the Water and Fire meridians.

- Kidney 1 (p.49)
- Heart 7 (p.48)
- Heart Protector 8 (p.50)

DEPRESSION

☞ Shiatsu can work well for depression.

☞ Give fairly strong Shiatsu with plenty of stretches and rotations for the Wood meridians.

- Liver 14 (p.51)
- Gall Bladder 21 (p.51)

INSOMNIA

☞ Gentle Shiatsu before bedtime is very successful.

☞ Work all the Fire meridians away from the head.

☞ Finish on the feet.

- Heart 7 (p.48)
- Heart Protector 6 (p.50)
- Kidney 1 (p.49)

NIGHT SWEATS

☞ Give deep Shiatsu to the Fire and Water meridians.

☞ If the night sweats persist consult a practitioner – Shiatsu usually helps.

- Bladder 23 (p.49)
- Kidney 7 (p.49)

STRESS

See Anxiety.

FATIGUE

☞ Shiatsu is excellent for tiredness and fatigue.

☞ Gentle Shiatsu on the Earth and Water meridians.

☞ Take plenty of time for self-Shiatsu.

- Stomach 36 (p.46)
- Spleen 6 (p.46)
- Bladder 23 (p.49)
- Kidney 1 (p.49)

HEADACHES

☞ Work on the face and head, and where the pain is. Then use the points below and finish with general work on the feet.

frontal headaches

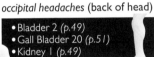

- Triple Heater 23 *(p.50)*
- Stomach 8 *(p.46)*
- Bladder 2 *(p.49)*

occipital headaches (back of head)

- Bladder 2 *(p.49)*
- Gall Bladder 20 *(p.51)*
- Kidney 1 *(p.49)*

one-sided headaches and migraine

- Triple Heater 23 *(p.50)*
- Gall Bladder 20 *(p.51)*
- Liver 3 *(p.51)*

NAUSEA

See Stomach-ache.

TRAVEL SICKNESS

See Morning sickness.

PAIN

☞ Pain anywhere in the body can be eased by holding the two points below. Hold one on the left hand and one on the right foot, and then swap over. Imagine a connection between the two points.

- Liver 3 *(p.51)*
- Large Intestine 4 *(p.47)*

NECK PROBLEMS

☞ Give a general Shiatsu to the face then gently draw the energy down the neck and give some deep Shiatsu to the shoulders. Continue to draw the energy out of the feet.

- Small Intestine 3 *(p.48)*
- Small Intestine 10 *(p.48)*
- Gall Bladder 20 *(p.51)*

SHOULDERS

☞ Give deep and firm Shiatsu to the shoulders, open the chest, and work with stretches and rotations.

☞ Work the stiffness out down the arms and out through the fingers.

- Small Intestine 3 *(p.48)*
- Small Intestine 10 *(p.48)*
- Gall Bladder 21 *(p.51)*

LOWER BACK PROBLEMS

☞ Working on the back and the Water meridians can often give relief.

☞ Pay attention to relaxing the buttocks. However, if there is further pain seek professional help.

- Bladder 23 *(p.49)*
- Kidney 1 *(p.49)*
- Kidney 3 *(p.49)*
- Small Intestine 3 *(p.48)*

KNEE PROBLEMS

☞ Firm Shiatsu on the Earth and Water meridians on the legs.

☞ Pay special attention to the knees, looking for needy areas around the kneecap and the back of the knee.

- Kidney 3 *(p.49)*
- Stomach 36 *(p.46)*

ARTHRITIS

☞ Shiatsu is very helpful for mobilizing joints which have become painful or stiff. Deep Shiatsu for the Water meridians followed by penetrating work on the actual joint. *See the section on Shiatsu for Water energy.*

MUSCLE CRAMPS

☞ Shiatsu works well.

☞ Work deeply on the affected area with slow stretches.

- Liver 3 *(p.51)*

MENSTRUAL PROBLEMS

☞ Work the abdomen and the lower back. Give Shiatsu to the Earth, Wood, and Water meridians, especially in the legs.

Flooding

- Spleen 6 *(p.46)*
- Kidney 3 *(p.49)*

Pain

- Spleen 6 *(p.46)*
- Liver 3 *(p.51)*

Absence of periods

- Kidney 3 *(p.49)*
- Spleen 6 *(p.46)*

Irregular

- Liver 3 *(p.51)*

MORNING SICKNESS

☞ First aid use of the point Heart Protector 6 (page 50) has been found to work in more than 50 per cent of women.

☞ It is possible to buy bands which will stimulate the point through the day. These are also sold as seasickness bands.

CHILDBIRTH – DURING LABOR

☞ Give firm Shiatsu on the shoulders and sacrum. Now is the time to use the points contraindicated in pregnancy.

- Large Intestine 4 *(p.47)*
- Gall Bladder 21 *(p.51)*
- Spleen 6 *(p.46)*

Further reading

A Practical Introduction: Shiatsu, by *Oliver Cowmeadow* (Element Books, 1998)

Bodymind Energetics, by *Mark Seem* (Thorsons, 1987)

Health Essentials: Shiatsu, by *Elaine Liechti* (Element Books, 1992)

Shiatsu Theory and Practice, by *Carola Beresford–Cooke* (Churchill Livingstone, 1966)

The Complete Illustrated Guide to Massage, by *Stewart Mitchell* (Element Books, 1997)

The Book of Shiatsu by *Lundberg* (Gaia, 1992)

Zen Shiatsu, by *Masunaga* (Japan Publications, 1977)

Useful addresses

American Oriental Bodywork Therapy Association
50 Maple Place
Manhasset NY 11030

The European Shiatsu Federation
Piazza S Agostino 24
20123 Milano
Italy

IMSV Shiatsu Association
Frans Copers
Zwarte Zustersstraat 30
B9000
Gent
Belgium

The Shiatsu Society (UK)
The Interchange Studios
Dalby Street
London NW5 3NQ

The Shiatsu Therapy Association of Australia
2 Caminoley Wynd
Templestowe 3106
Australia

Shiatsu Therapy Association of Ontario
PO Box 695
Station P
Toronto
Ontario M52Y4